DEFEATING THE SILENT INVADER(CANCER)

BUILDING A STRONGER IMMUNE SYSTEM AND OVERCOMING CANCER'S SURVIVAL TACTICS WITH THE RIGHT DIET AND LIFESTYLE CHOICES

DR GEORGE FEWELL

Copyright © 2023 [GEORGE FEWELL]

This book is intended to provide general information and does not constitute professional or expert advice. While every effort has been made to ensure the accuracy and completeness of the information contained in this book, the author, publisher, and any related parties assume no responsibility for errors or omissions or any damage or loss incurred due to the use of the information provided.

INTRODUCTION

Defeating the Silent Invader: Building a Stronger Immune System and Overcoming Cancer's Survival Tactics with the Right Diet and Lifestyle Choices" is a comprehensive guide penned by Dr. [George Fewell]. This book delves into the intricate relationship between the immune system, cancer, and the impact of diet and lifestyle choices on one's health.

At its core, the book aims to empower readers by offering a deeper understanding of how the immune system functions and its role in battling cancer cells. It shows how cancer cells evade the body's natural defenses and how a robust immune system can counteract these survival tactics.

Throughout the book, readers are given insights into the significance of adopting specific dietary patterns and lifestyle changes supporting immune health. The author presents a wealth of information, backed by scientific research, to illustrate how simple yet impactful alterations in diet and daily habits can positively influence immune function and potentially aid in overcoming cancer.

"Defeating the Silent Invader" is a beacon of hope for individuals seeking to comprehend the symbiotic relationship between their body's defenses, cancer, and the influence of lifestyle choices. It serves as a roadmap, offering practical advice and actionable steps to fortify the body's natural defenses and optimize overall health.

This book stands as a testament to the potential of informed decisions in creating a robust immune system and fostering an environment within the body that may contribute to overcoming the challenges posed by cancer.

In the subsequent chapters, the book delves into a myriad of topics, from exploring the pivotal role of nutrition in bolstering the immune system to unraveling the impact of stress management techniques on overall well-being. Each chapter is a treasure trove of knowledge, offering scientific insights, real-life anecdotes, and practical tips that readers can easily incorporate into their daily routines.

Moreover, "Defeating the Silent Invader" doesn't just focus on the theoretical aspects. It equips readers with actionable strategies, ranging from dietary adjustments and exercise regimens to mindfulness practices and holistic approaches, all designed to create an environment within the body that supports immune strength.

The author's approach is compassionate and scientifically grounded, catering to individuals seeking empowerment amidst their battle with cancer or those endeavoring to prevent its occurrence. The book instils a sense of control and optimism in the reader by demystifying the complex interplay between the immune system, cancer, and lifestyle choices.

As the chapters progress, "Defeating the Silent Invader" intricately weaves together the interconnected elements of diet, exercise, stress management, sleep hygiene, and environmental factors, elucidating their collective impact on immune function. It underscores the significance of a holistic approach, emphasizing that the synergy among these factors can potentiate the body's natural defenses against cancer and other health challenges.

Moreover, "Defeating the Silent Invader" doesn't only focus on battling cancer but also highlights the significance of preventive measures. It emphasizes that adopting a lifestyle geared towards immune support isn't solely about fighting disease—it's about nurturing overall well-being and resilience against various health challenges.

Ultimately, this book is a testament to the remarkable capacity of the human body to heal and thrive when provided with the right tools and environment. It stands as a comprehensive guide, offering hope, knowledge, and actionable steps toward building a more robust immune system and navigating the complex terrain of cancer with resilience and determination.

In the latter sections, "Defeating the Silent Invader" unveils the intricacies of the body's immune system, offering a deeper exploration into the mechanisms behind its response to cancer and how lifestyle interventions can tip the scales in favor of a healthier, more robust defense.

Furthermore, "Defeating the Silent Invader" doesn't limit itself to dietary suggestions; it provides a comprehensive understanding of how specific nutrients, antioxidants, and phytochemicals play a pivotal role in supporting immune function and potentially hindering cancer growth. It elucidates the power of food as medicine, offering a roadmap for incorporating immune-boosting foods and supplements into everyday life.

The book's holistic approach extends beyond individual choices to encompass the broader environmental factors influencing health. It sheds light on toxins, pollutants, and lifestyle factors that can compromise immune health, encouraging readers to create a nurturing environment that minimizes these detrimental influences.

In essence, "Defeating the Silent Invader" is not just a book about immune health and cancer—it's a holistic blueprint for living a life that nurtures the body, mind, and spirit. It empowers readers to embrace a proactive stance toward their health, offering a tapestry of knowledge, inspiration, and actionable strategies to unlock the body's innate potential for healing and resilience.

CHAPTER 1
❖THE NATURE OF CANCER CELLS

Cancer cells are characterized by their uncontrolled growth and division. Unlike normal cells that undergo a tightly regulated process of cell division, cancer cells divide continuously and rapidly, leading to the formation of tumors.

Cancer cells also can invade nearby tissues and spread to distant parts of the body through a process known as metastasis. This ability to spread and invade is one of the main reasons why cancer is so difficult to treat. Understanding the nature of cancer cells is crucial for developing effective treatments. Targeted therapies aim to specifically disrupt the unique features and mechanisms of cancer cells while sparing normal cells, thereby reducing side effects and improving treatment outcomes.

Cancer is a complex group of diseases characterized by the abnormal and uncontrolled growth of cells in the body. These cells divide and spread uncontrollably, forming tumors or affecting the blood and lymphatic systems.

Cancer isn't a single cause; it often results from a combination of genetic factors, environmental influences, and lifestyle choices. Mutations in the DNA can disrupt the normal functioning of cells, leading to unregulated growth. These mutations can be inherited or acquired during a person's lifetime due to exposure to carcinogens like tobacco smoke, UV radiation, certain chemicals, or viruses.

Cancer can affect any part of the body, and the type of cancer is typically named after the organ or tissue where it originates. There are more than 100 types of cancer, each with its characteristics, treatment options, and prognosis. Some common types include breast cancer, lung cancer, prostate cancer, colorectal cancer, and leukemia.

Treatment approaches for cancer depend on various factors, such as the type and stage of cancer, as well as the individual's overall health. Treatments may include surgery, chemotherapy, radiation therapy, immunotherapy, targeted therapy, hormone therapy, or a combination of these methods.

Early detection through screenings and adopting a healthy lifestyle with a balanced diet, regular exercise, avoiding tobacco, limiting alcohol consumption, and protecting oneself from harmful environmental factors can significantly reduce the risk of developing cancer. Research and advancements in medical science continue to improve our understanding and treatment of this complex disease.

❖UNVEILING CANCER'S STEALTH TACTICS

Cancer is a complex disease that involves the uncontrolled growth and spread of abnormal cells in the body. To survive and thrive, cancer cells have developed several stealth tactics that allow them to evade the body's immune system and resist traditional treatments. Unraveling these tactics is essential in developing effective strategies to combat cancer.

Here are some of cancer's stealth tactics:

IMMUNE EVASION:

Immune evasion is a strategy cancer cells use to avoid detection and destruction by the immune system. They can produce proteins that dampen the immune response or alter the expression of specific molecules on their surface, making them less recognizable as foreign by immune cells.

It is a crucial component of cancer progression and plays a significant role in tumor development and metastasis. Cancer cells evade the immune system by downregulating the expression of major histocompatibility complex (MHC) molecules on their surface.

MHC molecules present tumor antigens to immune cells, initiating an immune response against cancer cells. By reducing MHC expression, cancer cells escape recognition by immune cells, rendering the immune response ineffective.

Cancer cells also employ various mechanisms to avoid detection by immune cells. One such tool is inhibiting immune cell activation through the secretion of immunosuppressive cytokines and molecules. These molecules create an immunosuppressive microenvironment around the tumor, impairing the function of immune cells and preventing them from mounting an effective immune response against cancer.

Moreover, cancer cells can induce immune cell exhaustion, in which immune cells become dysfunctional and lose their ability to attack cancer cells. This exhaustion is caused by persistent stimulation and exposure to inhibitory signals generated by cancer cells. As a result, the immune cells become less responsive and fail to recognize and eliminate the cancer cells effectively.

In addition, cancer cells may undergo mutations in genes that are crucial for immune recognition. For example, mutations in the antigen-presenting machinery or cancer-specific surface antigens can lead to decreased recognition and attack by immune cells.

Furthermore, cancer cells can hijack immune checkpoint pathways to avoid immune surveillance. Immune checkpoints are regulatory molecules that prevent overactivation of the immune system and help maintain self-tolerance. However, cancer cells exploit these pathways by upregulating inhibitory checkpoints, such as programmed death-ligand 1 (PD-L1) or cytotoxic T-lymphocyte antigen 4 (CTLA-4), which bind to their corresponding receptors on immune cells, leading to their inactivation or suppression.

Understanding cancer cells' immune evasion mechanisms is critical for developing effective cancer immunotherapies. Targeting these immune evasion strategies, alone or in combination, can help restore and enhance the immune response against cancer cells, improving patient outcomes.

REPROGRAMMING OF THE MICROENVIRONMENT:

Reprogramming the microenvironment is a strategy cancer cells employ to evade detection and immune responses. The tumor microenvironment (TME) plays a crucial role in tumor development and progression, and cancer cells can exploit this environment to their advantage.

One way cancer cells reprogram the TME is by promoting an immunosuppressive environment. They can release cytokines, chemokines, and growth factors that suppress immune cells and impede their ability to recognize and eliminate cancer cells. By stopping the immune response, cancer cells can prevent the host immune system from recognizing them as foreign and evade immune surveillance.

Moreover, cancer cells remodel the extracellular matrix (ECM) within the TME to create a supportive environment for tumor growth. They can alter the composition and structure of the ECM, promoting invasion, metastasis, and angiogenesis. The modified ECM can also help shield cancer cells from immune cells and prevent them from reaching the tumor.

Additionally, cancer cells can manipulate the metabolism within the TME to their advantage. They can alter the availability of nutrients and oxygen, creating an inhospitable environment for immune cells and normal tissue cells while providing a selective advantage to cancer cells. By redirecting metabolic pathways, cancer cells can promote their survival and growth while impeding the function of immune cells.

Overall, reprogramming the microenvironment is a cancer stealth tactic that enables cancer cells to evade detection, immune responses, and therapeutic interventions. Understanding the mechanisms behind this reprogramming is essential for developing targeted therapies that disrupt the cancer cell-TME crosstalk and enhance anti-tumor immune responses.

DNA MUTATIONS AND GENOMIC INSTABILITY:

DNA mutations and genomic instability play a crucial role in cancer development and progression. Cancer cells often acquire and accumulate mutations in their DNA, leading to genomic instability. This instability enables cancer cells to evolve and adapt to their environment, making them highly elusive and difficult to target with conventional cancer therapies.

Cancer cells use DNA mutations and genomic instability as a stealth tactic by evading the immune system. The immune system is equipped to recognize and eliminate abnormal cells, including cancer cells. However, the genetic alterations in cancer cells can make them unrecognizable to the immune system, allowing them to go undetected and continue increasing.

Furthermore, DNA mutations and genomic instability contribute to cancer heterogeneity, meaning different cancer cells within a tumor can have distinct genetic profiles. This heterogeneity provides cancer cells with the ability to develop resistance to treatment and allows them to continue increasing even after therapy, leading to relapse and metastasis.

Additionally, genomic instability can lead to the activation of oncogenes, genes that can potentially transform normal cells into cancerous cells. These oncogenes can drive cancer cells' uncontrolled growth and division and promote their survival.

Cancer cells can acquire additional oncogenic alterations by continuously generating new mutations, further enhancing their survival and resistance to therapy.

Moreover, ongoing DNA mutations and genomic instability can lead to the loss of tumor suppressor genes, which usually inhibit cell growth and division. Losing these tumor suppressor genes allows cancer cells to escape regulatory mechanisms that prevent excessive cell proliferation, making them more elusive to treatment.

Overall, DNA mutations and genomic instability serve as a cancer stealth tactic by conferring cancer cells with the ability to evade the immune system, develop resistance to therapy, and adapt to different environments. Understanding and targeting these mutations and genomic instability pathways is crucial for developing effective cancer treatments to overcome these stealth tactics and improve patient outcomes.

METASTASIS:

Metastasis is a complex and fascinating process by which cancer cells spread from the primary tumor to other body parts. It is considered a significant challenge in cancer treatment and is responsible for the majority of cancer-related deaths.

One of the most intriguing aspects of metastasis is its ability to act as a stealth tactic. Cancer cells have developed various mechanisms to evade the immune system and establish themselves in distant organs, making them difficult to detect and eliminate.

Cancer cells undergo a series of genetic changes that enable them to detach from the original tumor mass and invade surrounding tissues. They can disguise themselves by altering the expression of cell surface molecules, which helps them evade recognition by immune cells. This allows them to blend in with normal cells and avoid immune system attacks.

Moreover, cancer cells can manipulate their microenvironment to create a favorable niche for survival and growth. They secrete signaling molecules that attract other cells and create a supportive environment for tumor progression. This includes releasing growth factors that promote blood vessel formation, allowing the tumor cells to receive nutrients and oxygen necessary for survival.

Additionally, cancer cells can undergo epithelial-to-mesenchymal transition (EMT), a process that alters their characteristics and enables them to acquire a more invasive and migratory phenotype. This transition makes them less susceptible to the immune system and allows them to navigate through the bloodstream or lymphatic system, reaching distant organs undetected.

Once they arrive at secondary sites, cancer cells can lie dormant for extended periods, escaping detection and potentially evading therapy. They can adapt to the novel microenvironment, establish new blood supply, and eventually form secondary tumors, contributing to the progression of the disease.

Understanding the mechanisms behind metastasis is vital for developing effective therapeutic strategies to target and eradicate disseminated cancer cells. By uncovering the cancer cells' stealth tactics, researchers can aim to develop approaches that disrupt their ability to metastasize and improve treatment outcomes for cancer patients.

RESISTANCE TO THERAPY:

Resistance to therapy is a phenomenon observed in various cancer patients, and it can be employed by cancer cells as a stealth tactic to evade the effects of treatment. Cancer cells are remarkably able to adapt and evolve, leading to resistance to commonly used therapies such as chemotherapy, targeted therapy, and immunotherapy. This resistance ultimately hampers the effectiveness of treatment and poses significant challenges to successful cancer management.

There are several mechanisms through which cancer cells can develop resistance. One mechanism involves genetic mutations or alterations that enable cancer cells to withstand the toxic effects of specific drugs. This can occur by acquiring gene mutations responsible for drug uptake, metabolism, and DNA repair or activating alternative signaling pathways to bypass the therapeutic target. In some cases, cancer cells may even develop efflux pumps that actively pump out drugs, reducing intracellular drug concentrations.

Additionally, the tumor microenvironment plays a crucial role in treatment resistance. Physical and molecular factors present in the surrounding tissues of the tumor can impede drug delivery or facilitate the growth and survival of therapy-resistant cancer cells. Factors such as hypoxia (lack of oxygen), high interstitial fluid pressure, and dense extracellular matrix can create a protective niche for resistant cells and impede the access of therapies to the tumor cells.

Resistance to therapy is a significant challenge in cancer treatment, as it not only reduces the effectiveness of initial therapy but also limits the options for subsequent treatments. Therefore, combating resistance requires a comprehensive understanding of the underlying mechanisms and the development of innovative therapeutic strategies.

Several approaches, such as combination therapies, are being explored, which involve targeting multiple pathways simultaneously to prevent the emergence of resistant populations. Additionally, research into novel therapeutic targets, the development of personalized medicine approaches, and immunotherapies are promising avenues to overcome therapy resistance.

Resistance to therapy serves as a cancer stealth tactic that allows tumor cells to survive and thrive despite treatment. Understanding the factors contributing to resistance and developing effective strategies are critical steps towards improving patient outcomes and ultimately winning the battle against cancer.

Understanding these stealth tactics of cancer is crucial for developing new treatment strategies.

❖THE ROLE OF THE IMMUNE SYSTEM

The immune system plays a crucial role in recognizing and eliminating cancer cells in the body.

Here are the fundamental mechanisms by which the immune system targets cancer cells:

IMMUNE SURVEILLANCE:

immune surveillance is a critical mechanism by which the immune system identifies and targets cancer cells in the body. It is a constant surveillance system that detects abnormal cells arising from genetic mutations and eliminates them before they can form a tumor.

The process of immune surveillance involves recognizing cancer cells as foreign or abnormal by immune cells, such as t cells and natural killer (nk) cells. These immune cells can identify specific markers, known as antigens, on the surface of cancer cells. These antigens can be derived from mutated or overexpressed proteins in cancer cells.

When cancer cells are identified, they initiate an immune response to eliminate them. T cells play a crucial role in immune surveillance by directly attacking and destroying cancer cells. They do this by releasing cytotoxic molecules, such as perforin and granzymes, which induce apoptosis (programmed cell death) in the cancer cells.

Nk cells also play a significant role in immune surveillance. They can recognize and directly kill cancer cells without prior sensitization, as they can detect alterations in surface markers commonly found on cancer cells.

Additionally, immune surveillance involves the production of pro-inflammatory cytokines by immune cells. These cytokines include interferons and interleukins, which can activate and recruit other immune cells to target and eliminate cancer cells.

While immune surveillance is an effective defense mechanism against cancer, there are cases where cancer cells can escape immune recognition. Some cancer cells develop strategies to evade immune detection by downregulating the expression of antigens or by secreting immunosuppressive factors. These mechanisms can weaken the immune response, allowing cancer cells to grow and spread.

Understanding the processes involved in immune surveillance has led to the development of various immunotherapies that aim to enhance the immune response against cancer. These treatments, such as immune checkpoint inhibitors and adoptive cell therapies, help overcome cancer cells' immune evasion strategies and improve immune surveillance.

Immune surveillance is a vital mechanism by which the immune system identifies and eliminates cancer cells. It involves the recognition of cancer cell antigens by t cells and nk cells, activating immune responses to eradicate the abnormal cells. Enhancing immune surveillance through immunotherapies has shown promising results in treating cancer.

T-CELL ACTIVATION:

T-cell activation is an essential mechanism by which the immune system targets cancer cells. T-cells, a white blood cell, play a crucial role in the adaptive immune response and are responsible for recognizing and eliminating cancer cells.

T-cell activation begins when t-cells recognize specific molecules, known as antigens, on the surface of cancer cells. These antigens can be derived from mutated or viral proteins expressed by the cancer cells. T-cells have t-cell receptors (tcrs) capable of binding to these antigens.

One crucial molecule released by activated t-cells is interferon-gamma (ifn-γ), which has several anti-cancer effects. Ifn-γ can increase the expression of molecules involved in antigen presentation on cancer cells, making them more easily recognizable by the immune system. It can also enhance the function of other immune cells, such as natural killer cells and macrophages, which can further contribute to eliminating cancer cells.

However, cancer cells have developed various mechanisms to evade t-cell activation and subsequent immune attack. They can downregulate the expression of antigens or molecules involved in antigen presentation, making them less recognizable by t-cells.

Additionally, cancer cells can produce immunosuppressive factors that inhibit t-cell activation and function, creating an immunosuppressive tumor microenvironment.

T-cell activation is a critical mechanism by which the immune system targets and eliminates cancer cells.

ANTIBODY-MEDIATED RESPONSE:

The antibody-mediated response is one of the mechanisms by which the immune system targets cancer cells. This response involves the production and activation of antibodies, which are y-shaped proteins that recognize and bind to specific molecules on cancer cells called antigens.

When cancer cells form in the body, they can express specific antigens on their surface that are not present in normal, healthy cells. These antigens can serve as targets for antibodies produced by the immune system. Antibodies are produced by a type of white blood cell called b cells, which can recognize and bind to specific antigens.

Once an antibody binds to an antigen on a cancer cell, it can trigger a cascade of immune responses. This can include activating other immune cells, such as natural killer (nk) cells or macrophages, which can kill or mark the cancer cells for destruction. Additionally, antibodies can activate the complement system, a group of proteins in the blood that can help destroy cancer cells.

In addition to their direct killing effects, antibodies can inhibit cancer cell growth and spread. They can block the signaling pathways that promote tumor cell survival and proliferation, or prevent the interaction of cancer cells with other cells in the body.

Furthermore, antibodies can recruit other immune cells to the site of the tumor through a process called antibody-dependent cellular cytotoxicity (adcc). This involves binding antibodies to cancer cells, which then attracts immune cells to destroy the tumor cells.

Scientists have developed several approaches to enhance the antibody-mediated immune response against cancer cells. This includes the development of monoclonal antibodies, which are laboratory-produced antibodies that target specific cancer antigens. These monoclonal antibodies can be used as therapeutic agents to target cancer cells or as vehicles to deliver drugs or radioactive substances directly to the tumor cells.

The antibody-mediated response is a crucial mechanism by which the immune system targets cancer cells. Understanding and manipulating this response holds great promise for developing effective immunotherapies against cancer.

NATURAL KILLER (NK) CELLS:

Natural killer (nk) cells, a type of white blood cell, play a crucial role in the body's immune system response against cancer cells. Nk cells are an integral part of the innate immune system and are designed to detect and eliminate abnormal cells, including cancer cells, without prior exposure or activation.

Nk cells are capable of recognizing and destroying cancer cells through various mechanisms. One of the primary ways is to detect specific receptors on the surface of cancer cells that distinguish them from healthy cells. These receptors allow nk cells to identify cancer cells as "non-self" or abnormal, triggering their activation.

Once activated, nk cells release cytotoxic granules containing perforin and granzymes that directly induce apoptosis (cell death) in the cancer cells. Moreover, nk cells can also regulate the immune response by secreting cytokines that enhance the activity of other immune cells, such as t cells, and promote an anti-tumor environment. Additionally, nk cells can coordinate with other immune cells to enhance the overall anti-cancer immune response.

While nk cells possess inherent cancer-fighting capabilities, various factors can hamper their effectiveness. Cancer cells often develop mechanisms to evade nk cell detection or suppress their function. For example, cancer cells can downregulate the surface expression of ligands that bind to nk cell receptors, making them less susceptible to recognition and attack. The tumor microenvironment may also create an immunosuppressive environment that can inhibit nk cell activity.

Researchers are actively studying ways to harness nk cells' potential in cancer immunotherapy. Strategies such as enhancing nk cell activity, genetically engineering nk cells to express specific receptors, or combining nk cell therapy with other immunotherapies are being explored to improve their efficacy in targeting and eradicating cancer cells.

In summary, nk cells are a vital mechanism through which the immune system targets cancer cells. Their ability to detect and eliminate abnormal cells and their role in enhancing the overall immune response highlights their immense potential in cancer immunotherapy. Ongoing research and advancements in this field hold promise for developing new therapeutic options to combat cancer.

IMMUNE MEMORY:

Immune memory is a crucial mechanism by which the immune system targets and destroys cancer cells. It refers to the ability of the immune system to remember a previous encounter with an antigen, enabling a faster and more robust immune response upon subsequent exposure.

When cancer cells develop in the body, they often express specific tumor antigens different from normal cells. The immune system recognizes these antigens as foreign and mounts an immune response to eliminate the cancer cells. During this process, specific immune cells, such as t and b cells, recognize and bind to the cancer antigens, destroying them.

After the initial encounter with cancer cells, a subset of t and b cells called memory cells are formed. These cells have a long lifespan and "remember" the particular tumor antigens they have encountered. If cancer cells reappear in the body, the memory cells can quickly identify the tumor antigens and initiate a more rapid and robust immune response.

Immune memory is crucial in cancer immunotherapy, particularly immune checkpoint blockade therapies. These therapies aim to enhance the immune system's ability to recognize and attack cancer cells. By blocking specific inhibitory signals in cancer cells or immune cells, these therapies activate memory cells and unleash a potent immune response against the tumor.

Additionally, immune memory contributes to the effectiveness of cancer vaccines. Vaccines containing specific tumor antigens can stimulate the immune system to generate memory cells that can recognize and target the cancer cells if they develop in the future.

Overall, immune memory is a vital factor in the immune system's ability to target cancer cells effectively. Harnessing and bolstering this mechanism through various therapeutic approaches is an active area of research in cancer immunology.

The immune system's ability to eliminate cancer cells can sometimes be compromised, leading to cancer progression. Enhancing the immune response against cancer cells, such as through immunotherapies like immune checkpoint inhibitors and adoptive cell therapy, has emerged as a promising approach in cancer treatment.

CHAPTER 2

❖STRENGTHENING THE BODY'S DEFENSES AGAINST CANCER CELLS

Cancer is a complex disease that occurs when abnormal cells divide and invade other tissues in the body. While various factors contribute to cancer development, maintaining a robust immune system can help strengthen the body's defenses against cancer cells.

Here are some notes on how to strengthen the body's defenses against cancer cells:

REGULAR EXERCISE:

Regular exercise has been shown to have numerous benefits for overall health, including its potential to strengthen the body's defenses against cancer cells.

Exercise helps to boost the immune system, which plays a crucial role in identifying and eliminating cancer cells. It promotes the production of various immune cells, such as natural killer cells, T cells, and macrophages, responsible for detecting and destroying abnormal cells, including cancer cells.

Furthermore, exercise helps to control body weight and reduce obesity, which is a significant risk factor for several types of cancer, including breast, colorectal, and endometrial cancer. Maintaining a healthy weight through exercise can help minimize cancer cell development.

Regular physical activity also aids in reducing inflammation throughout the body. Chronic inflammation has been linked to the development and progression of various cancers. By decreasing inflammation levels, exercise helps to create an environment less conducive to cancer cell formation.

Moreover, exercise has been found to enhance the body's utilization of insulin and improve insulin sensitivity. This is important as elevated insulin levels have been associated with an increased risk of developing certain types of cancer, such as breast, colon, and pancreatic cancer.

In addition to these direct benefits, exercise indirectly strengthens the body's defenses against cancer by reducing stress levels.

Chronic stress has been linked to the weakening of the immune system and the promotion of tumor growth. Regular exercise helps manage stress and improve mental well-being, thereby indirectly improving the body's ability to fight off cancer cells.

It's important to note that while exercise can provide significant health benefits and potentially reduce the risk of cancer, it should not be considered a standalone cancer treatment. Regular exercise should be combined with a healthy lifestyle, such as a balanced diet, adequate rest, and avoiding harmful behaviors like smoking and excessive alcohol consumption, to maximize its effect on cancer prevention.

ANTIOXIDANT-RICH FOODS:

Antioxidants are natural compounds in plants, fruits, vegetables, and other food sources. They protect the body's cells from damage caused by harmful molecules called free radicals produced during normal cellular processes and exposure to environmental factors such as pollution, radiation, or smoking. By neutralizing these free radicals, antioxidants prevent them from causing damage to the DNA and other vital components of our cells, reducing the risk of developing cancer.

Many antioxidants have been studied for their potential anti-cancer properties. Some commonly known ones include vitamins A, C, and E and minerals like selenium and zinc. Other plant compounds such as flavonoids, polyphenols, and carotenoids have also shown promising effects in combating cancer.

Various studies have linked a diet rich in antioxidant-containing foods with a reduced risk of several types of cancers, including lung, breast, prostate, and colorectal cancers, among others. These foods include berries, dark leafy greens, citrus fruits, nuts, seeds, tomatoes, cruciferous vegetables (broccoli, cauliflower, cabbage), and green tea.

While a diet high in antioxidant-rich foods is beneficial, it is essential to note that it should not be considered a stand-alone cancer prevention or treatment method. It is always recommended to combine a balanced diet with other healthy lifestyle choices, such as regular exercise, avoiding tobacco and excessive alcohol consumption, and maintaining a healthy body weight.

Furthermore, consulting with healthcare professionals regarding individual dietary needs and any existing medical conditions is crucial. They can provide personalized guidance and treatment plans tailored to specific circumstances, including cancer prevention or management.

Consuming a diet rich in antioxidant-containing foods can be a helpful strategy to strengthen the body's defenses against cancer cells.

CANCER-FIGHTING FOODS:

Cancer-fighting foods are widely recognized as valuable to a healthy diet to boost the body's defenses against cancer cells. While no single food can prevent or cure cancer, incorporating specific foods into our meals can provide essential nutrients and compounds that support our immune system and fight against cancer cells.

Here are some critical points to note about cancer-fighting foods:

1. Antioxidant-rich fruits and vegetables: Plant-based foods are high in antioxidants, which help neutralize free radicals that can damage DNA and lead to cancer development. Include a variety of colorful fruits and vegetables like berries, leafy greens, cruciferous vegetables (e.g., broccoli, cabbage), and citrus fruits in your diet.

2. Fiber-packed whole grains: Whole grains like brown rice, quinoa, and whole wheat provide essential fiber, which aids in digestion, helps maintain a healthy weight, and reduces the risk of colorectal cancer. Replace refined grains with whole grains whenever possible.

3. Cruciferous vegetables: Cruciferous vegetables contain various compounds that may help prevent cancer. For example, broccoli, cauliflower, and Brussels sprouts are rich in sulforaphane, which has been found to inhibit the growth of cancer cells and reduce the risk of several types of cancer, including breast, lung, and colorectal cancer.

4. Healthy fats: Opt for healthy fats that promote overall well-being, such as avocados, nuts, seeds, and olive oil. These fats provide essential nutrients and are associated with a lower risk of certain cancers, such as breast and prostate cancer.

5. Omega-3 fatty acids: Fatty fish, such as salmon, mackerel, and sardines, are excellent sources of omega-3 fatty acids, which have anti-inflammatory properties and may help reduce the risk of various cancers, including breast, prostate, and colorectal cancer. If you don't consume fish, consider incorporating plant-based sources like chia seeds, flaxseeds, and walnuts.

6. Green tea: Green tea contains polyphenols, which are believed to have antioxidant and anti-inflammatory properties. Regular consumption of green tea has been linked to a reduced risk of several cancers, including breast, prostate, and colorectal cancer. Enjoy a cup or two of green tea daily as a healthy diet.

7. Spices and herbs: Many spices and herbs, like turmeric, ginger, garlic, and cinnamon, possess antioxidant and anti-inflammatory properties. Incorporating them into your meals adds flavor and provides potential cancer-fighting benefits.

Remember that maintaining a well-balanced diet, regular physical activity, avoiding tobacco products, limiting alcohol consumption, and staying healthy are all critical factors in reducing cancer risk. Always consult a healthcare professional for personalized nutrition advice and ensure a well-rounded approach to cancer prevention and treatment.

REGULAR SCREENING:

Regular screening is essential for strengthening the body's defenses against cancer cells. It plays a crucial role in early detection and prevention, allowing for timely intervention and increased chances of successful treatment.

Screening tests can help identify cancer cells or abnormal changes in the body before they cause noticeable symptoms. Detecting cancer early can initiate treatment promptly, improving the chances of a favorable outcome. Moreover, some screenings, such as mammograms and Pap tests, are specifically designed to detect precancerous conditions, enabling preventive measures to be taken before cancer develops.

Regular screening is essential for individuals who have inherited genetic mutations associated with cancer or have a family history of the disease. These individuals often have a higher risk of developing cancer and can benefit significantly from early detection and proactive management.

While screening tests are practical, they do have limitations. False positives and false negatives can occur, leading to unnecessary anxiety or delayed diagnosis, respectively. However, healthcare providers consider these factors and use a combination of different screening methods to increase accuracy and reduce the risk of false results.

Moreover, screening should be complemented by a healthy lifestyle and risk-reducing behaviors. This includes maintaining a balanced diet, engaging in regular physical activity, avoiding tobacco and excessive alcohol consumption, and protecting oneself from known carcinogens.

Regular screening is crucial in strengthening the body's defenses against cancer cells. It enables early detection, facilitates timely treatment, and ultimately improves the chances of successful outcomes. Regular medical check-ups and cancer screenings can detect cancer at an early stage when treatment is often more effective.

STRESS MANAGEMENT:

Stress management is vital in strengthening the body's defenses against cancer cells. It is well-known that chronic stress weakens the immune system, making individuals more susceptible to various diseases, including cancer. Therefore, adopting effective stress management techniques can significantly improve overall health and enhance the body's ability to fight cancer.

One of the primary ways stress management helps strengthen the body's defenses against cancer is by reducing stress hormones like cortisol. When stress hormones are consistently elevated, they hinder the immune system's ability to identify and destroy cancer cells. By practicing stress management techniques such as meditation, deep breathing exercises, or engaging in hobbies, individuals can lower stress hormone levels and thus support a healthier immune response against cancer.

Moreover, stress management positively influences lifestyle factors that are closely associated with cancer prevention and treatment. High-stress levels often lead to unhealthy coping mechanisms like overeating, smoking, or excessive alcohol consumption.

These behaviors not only weaken the immune system but also increase the risk of developing cancer. By managing stress effectively, individuals are more likely to adopt healthier habits, such as maintaining a balanced diet, exercising regularly, and avoiding harmful substances. These health-promoting behaviors create a more hostile environment for cancer cells, making it more challenging for them to survive and proliferate.

Furthermore, stress management techniques help improve mental and emotional well-being, indirectly contributing to cancer prevention and treatment. Chronic stress can lead to depression, anxiety, and sleep disturbances, all of which negatively impact the immune system's functioning and can promote cancer growth. By reducing stress levels and improving mental health through techniques like mindfulness or therapy, individuals can create a positive mindset, enhance resilience, and increase the effectiveness of cancer treatments.

Here are some practical ways to effectively manage stress:

1. Maintain a healthy lifestyle: Adopt a balanced diet, exercise regularly, and get sufficient sleep. These lifestyle choices can help reduce stress and improve overall well-being.

2. Practice relaxation techniques: Incorporate relaxation techniques such as deep breathing exercises, mindfulness meditation, yoga, or tai chi into your daily routine. These techniques promote relaxation and reduce stress levels.

3. Stay socially connected: Build a robust support system by maintaining relationships with friends, family, or support groups. Talking to others about your concerns can help alleviate stress and provide emotional support.

4. Manage time effectively: Prioritize tasks, set realistic goals, and avoid overcommitting yourself. Time management techniques can reduce stress by creating a sense of control over your schedule.

5. Engage in hobbies and activities you enjoy: Participate in activities that bring you joy and help you relax, such as hobbies, sports, reading, or listening to music. These activities can distract from stressors and provide a sense of fulfillment.

6. Practice self-care: Take time for yourself by engaging in activities that promote self-care and self-compassion. This can include taking a bath, practicing mindfulness, getting a massage, or indulging in a hobby you enjoy.

7. Seek support from professionals: If stress becomes overwhelming, consider seeking the help of a mental health professional. They can provide guidance and support in coping with stress, anxiety, and any emotional challenges related to cancer prevention.

Managing stress is crucial for maintaining good overall health and reducing cancer risk. It is important to prioritize self-care and adopt strategies that work best for you.

Stress management is essential to strengthening the body's defenses against cancer cells. By reducing stress hormone levels, adopting healthy habits, and improving mental well-being, individuals can create an unfavorable environment for cancer growth and bolster their immune system's ability to combat cancer. Therefore, incorporating stress management techniques into daily life is crucial for cancer prevention, treatment, and overall well-being.

ENVIRONMENTAL INTELLIGENCE:

Environmental intelligence refers to the knowledge and understanding of the environment and its impact on human health. It is crucial in promoting a healthy lifestyle and can help strengthen the body's defenses against cancer cells.

Cancer is a complex disease influenced by various factors, including genetic predisposition, lifestyle choices, and environmental exposures. By harnessing environmental intelligence, individuals can make informed decisions to create a healthier living environment and minimize potential risks associated with cancer.

Here are a few ways in which environmental intelligence can contribute to strengthening the body's defenses against cancer cells:

1. Avoiding environmental carcinogens: Environmental intelligence helps identify and avoid potential carcinogens present in our surroundings. It allows individuals to be aware of harmful substances such as tobacco smoke, pesticides, industrial chemicals, and air pollutants that may increase cancer risk. Individuals can significantly reduce their cancer risk by taking measures to minimize exposure to these carcinogens.

2. Promoting a healthy diet: Environmental intelligence emphasizes the importance of a balanced and nutritious diet. It educates individuals about the benefits of consuming organic and locally sourced foods, which are generally free from harmful pesticides and chemicals. Individuals can enhance their immune systems and reduce cancer risk by making healthier choices and avoiding processed or high-fat foods.

3. Creating a non-toxic living environment: Environmental intelligence encourages individuals to create a non-toxic environment using eco-friendly cleaning products, personal care items, and household items. This helps to reduce exposure to potentially carcinogenic substances present in traditional products. By opting for non-toxic alternatives, individuals can create a safer environment for themselves and their families, reducing the risk of cancer.

4. Practicing safe sun exposure: Environmental intelligence educates individuals about the harmful effects of excessive sun exposure and the importance of using sunscreen and protective clothing to prevent skin cancer. By following safe sun practices, such as avoiding peak sunlight hours and using broad-spectrum sunscreen, individuals can protect their skin and lower the risk of developing skin cancer.

Incorporating environmental intelligence into our daily lives can lead to a healthier lifestyle and strengthen the body's defenses against cancer cells. By being aware of our surroundings and making informed choices, we can create an environment that promotes well-being and reduces cancer risk.

Environmental intelligence strengthens the body's defenses against cancer cells. By improving recognition and response to potential carcinogens, activating the immune system, and supporting detoxification mechanisms, individuals can enhance their ability to prevent and combat the development of cancer cells. Adopting a healthy lifestyle and managing stress are vital to maintaining optimal environmental intelligence and reducing cancer risk.

EARLY DETECTION AND TREATMENT: Early detection and treatment are crucial in strengthening the body's defenses against cancer cells. Detecting cancer at an early stage significantly increases the chances of successful treatment and improves overall prognosis.

Regular screenings and medical check-ups help identify cancerous cells in their early stages, even before any noticeable symptoms arise. Early detection enables doctors to intervene quickly and employ suitable treatment options such as surgery, radiation therapy, chemotherapy, or immunotherapy. By starting treatment early, doctors can prevent the spread of cancer cells to other parts of the body and potentially eliminate or reduce the size of the tumor.

Moreover, early treatment can enhance the body's immune response against cancer cells. Specific therapies, like immunotherapy, help stimulate the immune system, making it more effective in recognizing and destroying cancer cells. Immunotherapy has shown promising results in various types of cancers, and when used in combination with early detection, it can improve outcomes significantly.

Early detection and prompt treatment also prevent cancer from causing severe damage to vital organs. Cancer cells can invade nearby tissues and organs, interfering with proper functioning. Detecting and treating cancer early minimizes the potential for long-term wear.

Additionally, early detection allows patients to adopt a proactive approach towards their health. It enables them to make lifestyle modifications, such as quitting smoking, maintaining a healthy weight, exercising regularly, and consuming a balanced diet. These lifestyle changes contribute to overall well-being and support the body's defenses against cancer cells.

Early detection and treatment are critical strategies in strengthening the body's defenses against cancer cells. It allows for timely intervention, improving treatment outcomes and reducing the impact on the body's organs.

CHAPTER 3
❖OPTIMIZING DIET FOR RESILIENCE

Optimizing diet for resilience involves making choices that support overall health and well-being, bolstering the body's ability to cope with stress, adapt to life's challenges, and bounce back from adversity.

Optimizing your diet for resilience against cancer involves making confident dietary choices that can help prevent the development and progression of cancer cells in the body.

Here are some key recommendations:

INCLUDE A VARIETY OF FRUITS AND VEGETABLES:

Eating a diet rich in various fruits and vegetables are vital for optimizing resilience against cancer. These natural foods contain many nutrients, antioxidants, and phytochemicals proven to have anti-cancer properties.

Here are some key points to consider when incorporating fruits and vegetables into your diet for cancer prevention:

1. Aim for a Rainbow of Colors: Consume fruits and vegetables of different colors daily. Each hue represents different beneficial plant compounds that can protect against various forms of cancer. Include red tomatoes, blueberries, orange carrots, leafy greens, purple grapes, yellow bell peppers, and more to ensure a diverse nutrient intake.

2. Emphasize Cruciferous Vegetables: Cruciferous vegetables like broccoli, cauliflower, Brussels sprouts, and kale contain sulfur compounds that enhance the body's detoxification processes and reduce cancer risk. Aim for several servings of cruciferous vegetables each week.

3. Consume Berries Regularly: Berries, such as strawberries, raspberries, blueberries, and blackberries, are packed with antioxidants and phytochemicals that help neutralize free radicals and reduce inflammation, which is crucial for cancer prevention.

4. Include Citrus Fruits: Citrus fruits like oranges, lemons, limes, and grapefruits are excellent sources of vitamin C and other antioxidants. These nutrients act as powerful immune boosters and aid in preventing DNA damage caused by cancer-causing agents.

5. Don't Forget Allium Vegetables: Allium vegetables like garlic, onions, leeks, and shallots contain compounds that have been shown to inhibit the growth of cancer cells. They also have immune-enhancing and anti-inflammatory properties.

6. Leafy Greens are Essential: Dark leafy greens like spinach, kale, Swiss chard, and collard greens are loaded with vitamins, minerals, and fiber. They contain various cancer-fighting compounds and benefit overall health and cancer prevention.

7. Variety is Key: Incorporate a wide variety of fruits and vegetables into your diet to ensure you receive a broad range of nutrients and antioxidants. Experiment with different recipes and include seasonal produce to keep your meals exciting and satisfying.

Remember, while a diet rich in fruits and vegetables is essential for cancer prevention, it should complement other healthy lifestyle choices such as regular exercise, reducing stress, limiting processed foods, and avoiding tobacco and excessive alcohol consumption.

CHOOSE WHOLE GRAINS:

Choosing whole grains as a means of optimizing diet for resilience against cancer is an intelligent and proactive approach. There are several reasons why whole grains are beneficial in reducing the risk of cancer and promoting overall health:

1. High in Fiber: Whole grains are an excellent source of dietary fiber, which plays a crucial role in maintaining a healthy digestive system. Fiber aids in regular bowel movements prevents constipation and reduces the risk of colorectal cancer. It also helps regulate blood sugar levels, keeping them stable and reducing the risk of developing type 2 diabetes, associated with an increased risk of certain cancers.

2. Rich in Antioxidants: Whole grains contain various antioxidants, including phenolic compounds, lignans, and vitamin E. These antioxidants help neutralize harmful free radicals in the body, which can cause cell damage and lead to cancer development. Studies have shown that a diet high in antioxidants can reduce the risk of various cancers, including breast, colon, and prostate.

3. Lower Glycemic Index: Whole grains have a lower glycemic index than refined grains. This means they are digested more slowly, providing a steady release of energy and preventing spikes in blood sugar levels. High glycemic index foods, such as refined grains and sugar, have been linked to an increased risk of certain cancers, particularly pancreatic and endometrial cancer.

4. Nutrient Dense: Whole grains contain essential nutrients such as B-vitamins, minerals (iron, magnesium, selenium), and phytochemicals. These nutrients play crucial roles in maintaining a healthy immune system, promoting DNA repair, and preventing cellular damage, all contributing to cancer prevention.

Opt for whole wheat, brown rice, quinoa, oats, barley, and millet when choosing whole grains. Incorporating these into your diet can be easy and delicious. Swap refined grains (such as white bread and white rice) with whole grain options, include whole grain cereals or oatmeal in your breakfast, and experiment with different whole grain-based recipes.

It is important to note that while whole grains offer many benefits, they should be part of a balanced and varied diet. It is also essential to consult with a healthcare professional or a registered dietitian to tailor your diet to your specific needs and incorporate other cancer-preventive foods such as fruits, vegetables, lean proteins, and healthy fats. Remember, diet alone cannot guarantee immunity against cancer, but it can be essential to an overall healthy lifestyle.

LIMIT PROCESSED AND RED MEATS:

Eating a balanced and varied diet is crucial for overall health, including reducing cancer risk. One important aspect to consider is the consumption of processed and red meats, as they have been linked to an increased risk of certain types of cancer, particularly colorectal cancer.

Processed meats are products modified through salting, curing, fermentation, or other processes to enhance flavor or improve preservation. These include sausages, hot dogs, bacon, ham, and certain deli meats. On the other hand, red meats include beef, pork, lamb, and goat.

Research has shown that consuming processed meats regularly can increase the risk of developing colorectal cancer. The World Health Organization's International Agency for Research on Cancer (IARC) classifies processed meats as Group 1 carcinogens, which means they are known to cause cancer in humans. Red meats are classified as Group 2A, meaning they are probably carcinogenic to humans.

Limiting the consumption of processed and red meats is recommended to optimize your diet for resilience against cancer. Instead, include other protein sources in your diet, such as poultry, fish, legumes, nuts, and seeds. Plant-based protein sources often contain additional nutrients like fiber, vitamins, and minerals that can also contribute to reducing cancer risks.

Moreover, increasing the intake of fruits, vegetables, and whole grains can provide protective compounds, such as antioxidants and phytochemicals, which help fight against cancer. These foods offer a wide range of nutrients and fiber, supporting overall health and boosting the body's resilience against cancer.

Additionally, maintaining a healthy weight, being physically active, limiting alcohol consumption, quitting smoking, and reducing exposure to environmental carcinogens are all critical factors in optimizing your diet for resilience against cancer. Remember, it is always best to consult with a healthcare professional or a registered dietitian to receive personalized dietary advice based on your needs and health conditions.

INCLUDE HEALTHY FATS:

Including healthy fats in the diet can be a valuable component in optimizing resilience against cancer. While it is important to note that diet alone cannot prevent or cure cancer, a well-balanced diet that includes healthy fats can support overall health and reduce the risk of developing certain types of cancer.

Healthy fats, such as monounsaturated and polyunsaturated fats, are vital for the body's optimal functioning and can provide various benefits when included in the diet.

Here are some reasons why healthy fats are beneficial for resilience against cancer:

1. Anti-inflammatory properties: Chronic inflammation increases the risk of developing cancer. Healthy fats, such as those found in avocados, olive oil, fatty fish, nuts, and seeds, contain anti-inflammatory compounds that can help reduce inflammation.

2. Nutrient absorption: Certain vitamins and minerals, such as vitamins A, D, E, and K, are fat-soluble, meaning they require the presence of fat to be adequately absorbed by the body. Including healthy fats alongside nutrient-rich foods can enhance the absorption of these essential nutrients.

3. Cell protection: Healthy fats, specifically omega-3 fatty acids found in fatty fish like salmon and chia seeds, have been linked to protecting cellular health and reducing the risk of various types of cancer, including colorectal and breast cancer.

4. Energy source: Fats are a concentrated energy source that can sustain energy levels throughout the day. Including healthy fats can help maintain a healthy weight and reduce the risk of obesity, a known risk factor for various types of cancer.

5. Hormonal balance: Some types of cancer, such as hormone-related cancers like breast and prostate cancer, are influenced by certain hormone levels in the body. Healthy fats can help regulate hormone production and balance hormonal levels, reducing the risk of hormone-related cancers.

It is important to note that not all fats are created equal, and it is essential to choose healthy fats over unhealthy ones, such as saturated and trans fats, which can increase inflammation and the risk of chronic diseases, including cancer.

Incorporating healthy fats into a well-balanced diet is a vital strategy to optimize resilience against cancer. They provide anti-inflammatory properties, aid nutrient absorption, protect cellular health, supply energy, and promote hormonal balance. However, consulting with a healthcare professional or a registered dietitian for personalized dietary advice tailored to your specific needs is always recommended. These fats contain antioxidants and anti-inflammatory properties that may help prevent cancer development.

STAY HYDRATED:

Staying hydrated is often overlooked but is an essential aspect of optimizing your diet for resilience against cancer. Adequate hydration is crucial for overall health and plays a significant role in cancer prevention and treatment.

Here are some key points to consider:

1. Water is essential: Our bodies comprise about 60% water, which involves numerous bodily functions. Water helps transport nutrients to cells, eliminate waste products, regulate body temperature, and maintain proper organ function.

2. Flushes out toxins: Proper hydration assists in flushing out harmful toxins and waste products from our bodies. This reduces the risk of accumulating toxins that may damage cells and lead to cancer development.

3. Supports healthy cell function: Water plays a pivotal role in maintaining the health and function of our cells. Well-hydrated cells are more resilient and have an improved ability to repair DNA damage, which is crucial for preventing cancerous cell growth.

4. Promotes digestion and nutrient absorption: Staying hydrated aids in proper digestion and the absorption of essential nutrients. This ensures that your body can effectively utilize the nutrients from the foods you consume, promoting overall well-being and resilience against cancer.

5. Helps with the side effects of cancer treatments: Many cancer treatments, such as chemotherapy, can cause dehydration as a side effect. Adequate hydration during treatment helps alleviate symptoms like fatigue, nausea, and constipation, optimizing overall recovery and resilience.

TO STAY HYDRATED AND OPTIMIZE YOUR DIET FOR RESILIENCE AGAINST CANCER, FOLLOW THESE TIPS:

- Drink plenty of water throughout the day. Aim for at least 8 glasses (64 ounces) or more, depending on your needs and activity level.

- Limit or avoid sugary drinks, as they can contribute to inflammation and an increased risk of cancer.

- Consume hydrating foods such as fruits and vegetables with high water content. Examples include watermelon, cucumbers, oranges, and strawberries.

- Avoid excessive caffeine and alcohol consumption, as they can dehydrate your body.

- Monitor your urine color - clear or light-yellow urine indicates good hydration.

- Be mindful of your hydration needs during hot weather, strenuous activities, or when undergoing cancer treatments.

Remember, staying hydrated is just one piece of the puzzle in maintaining a well-balanced and cancer-resilient diet. Incorporate various nutrient-dense foods, maintain a healthy weight, engage in regular physical activity, and consult a healthcare professional for personalized dietary recommendations.

It's essential to note that while diet plays a significant role in cancer prevention, it is not a foolproof method. Regular screenings, exercise, maintaining a healthy lifestyle, and avoiding tobacco are also crucial for reducing cancer risk. Consult with a healthcare professional or registered dietitian for personalized dietary recommendations based on your needs and medical history.

❖ EFFECT OF PHYTOCHEMICALS IN CANCER PREVENTION AND CONTROL

Phytochemicals are naturally occurring compounds found in plants, and research has shown that they have various health benefits, including cancer prevention and treatment.

Here are some effects of phytochemicals in cancer prevention and control:

ANTIOXIDANT ACTIVITY:

Antioxidants help protect cells from damage caused by harmful molecules called free radicals. Free radicals are highly reactive and can damage cell structures, including DNA, proteins, and lipids. This damage can lead to the development and progression of cancer.

Phytochemicals have been found to have potent antioxidant properties. They are capable of neutralizing free radicals and preventing oxidative damage to cells. This antioxidant activity is believed to be one of the main mechanisms by which phytochemicals can help prevent and control cancer.

There are several ways in which phytochemicals exert their antioxidant effects. They can directly scavenge and neutralize free radicals, preventing them from damaging cells. Phytochemicals can also stimulate the body's antioxidant defense mechanisms, such as increasing the production of endogenous antioxidants like glutathione and superoxide dismutase.

Furthermore, phytochemicals can inhibit the activity of enzymes that are involved in the production of free radicals. For example, some phytochemicals can inhibit the enzyme cyclooxygenase, which is involved in producing reactive oxygen species.

Numerous studies have shown that phytochemicals with antioxidant activity, such as flavonoids, phenols, and carotenoids, have cancer-preventive effects. They have been found to inhibit the growth and division of cancer cells, induce apoptosis (programmed cell death) in cancer cells, and inhibit the formation of new blood vessels necessary for tumor growth.

ANTI-INFLAMMATORY EFFECTS:

Chronic inflammation is linked to the development and progression of cancer. Inflammation is a complex biological process that plays a role in the development and progression of cancer. Chronic inflammation can lead to DNA damage, cell proliferation, and angiogenesis, all of which are hallmarks of cancer.

Numerous studies have shown that phytochemicals can help modulate the inflammatory response in the body. These compounds can inhibit the production of pro-inflammatory molecules, such as cytokines, prostaglandins, and nitric oxide, while promoting the production of anti-inflammatory molecules. Doing so, they help maintain a balance in the immune system and limits excessive inflammatory responses.

Many phytochemicals have been found to possess anti-inflammatory properties, including curcumin from turmeric, resveratrol from grapes, lycopene from tomatoes, and flavonoids found in fruits and vegetables. These compounds can target various signaling pathways involved in inflammation, such as NF-κB, MAPK, and COX-2.

By reducing inflammation, phytochemicals may help prevent the initiation and progression of cancer. Inflammation creates a favorable environment for the growth and survival of cancer cells. It can promote the formation of tumors, enhance angiogenesis, and facilitate the spread of cancer cells. By attenuating the inflammatory response, phytochemicals can potentially inhibit these processes and limit the growth and spread of cancer cells.

In addition to their anti-inflammatory effects, phytochemicals also exert other beneficial effects on cancer prevention and control. They can induce apoptosis (programmed cell death), inhibit cell proliferation, and suppress metastasis. Moreover, some phytochemicals have antioxidant properties, protecting cells from oxidative damage and reducing the risk of DNA mutations.

HORMONAL REGULATION:

Several phytochemicals have been found to possess hormone-regulating properties. For instance, isoflavones, a type of phytoestrogen found in soybeans and other legumes, can exert estrogenic or antiestrogenic effects depending on the hormonal background. By binding to estrogen receptors, isoflavones can regulate estrogen levels and prevent the adverse effects associated with excess estrogen, such as breast and endometrial cancers.

Similarly, other phytochemicals like indoles found in cruciferous vegetables, such as broccoli and cabbage, can influence estrogen metabolism, decreasing the production of harmful forms of estrogen that contribute to cancer development.

These indole compounds also can inhibit the activity of enzymes involved in estrogen synthesis, further regulating hormone levels.

Additionally, phytochemicals like lignans and resveratrol found in flaxseeds, whole grains, and red grapes respectively, have been shown to have antiestrogenic effects, reducing the risk of hormone-dependent cancers. They can bind to estrogen receptors, competing with endogenous estrogen and limiting its proliferative effects on cancer cells.

Furthermore, phytochemicals can also influence other hormones, such as androgens, which play a role in the development of prostate cancer.

For example, lycopene, a carotenoid compound found in tomatoes, has been associated with lower prostate cancer risk. It is believed to inhibit the production of androgens and decrease the expression of androgen receptors, thus helping to regulate hormone levels and prevent the growth of prostate cancer cells.

INHIBITION OF CANCER CELL GROWTH: Several phytochemicals, such as polyphenols, flavonoids, carotenoids, and glycosylates, have been extensively studied for their anticancer properties. For example, resveratrol has been shown to inhibit the growth of various cancer cells, including breast, prostate, and colorectal.

These compounds possess various mechanisms that contribute to their ability to inhibit cancer cell growth. For instance, they can interfere with key signaling pathways in cell proliferation, induce apoptosis (programmed cell death), inhibit angiogenesis (formation of blood vessels that supply tumors), and exert anti-inflammatory effects.

One of the essential characteristics of phytochemicals is their ability to simultaneously target multiple cancer-related processes, a property lacking in many traditional cancer therapies. These compounds have been shown to selectively target cancer cells while leaving normal cells unharmed, which reduces the adverse effects common to conventional cancer treatments.

Phytochemicals demonstrate synergistic effects when consumed in whole foods or as combinations, indicating that their beneficial effects are likely due to the combined actions of various compounds working together.

ENHANCEMENT OF IMMUNE FUNCTION: Phytochemicals can have immunomodulating effects, enhancing the immune system's function. Phytochemicals can help boost the immune response against cancer cells by stimulating immune cells, modulating inflammatory responses, and enhancing the overall immune function. For example, some phytochemicals have been found to increase the production of natural killer (NK) cells, which are critical in recognizing and killing cancer cells.

Additionally, phytochemicals can regulate the production and activity of various immune cells, such as T cells and macrophages, improving their ability to remove cancerous cells. These compounds can also reduce the production of pro-inflammatory cytokines that promote tumor growth and metastasis.

Moreover, phytochemicals possess antioxidant properties, protecting immune cells from oxidative damage caused by free radicals. This protection helps to maintain the optimal functioning of immune cells and their ability to fight against cancer cells.

Studies have demonstrated the potential of phytochemicals in enhancing immune function and reducing the risk of cancer development and progression. However, it's important to note that the effects of phytochemicals on immune function may vary depending on the specific compound and dosage used, as well as individual differences in metabolism and genetics.

CHAPTER 4
❖OVERCOMING CHALLENGES AND SUSTAINING HOPE

The journey of cancer prevention and control often presents numerous challenges that individuals and their loved ones must navigate. From the physical and emotional tolls of treatment to the financial burden and the fear of recurrence, it can be an incredibly difficult and overwhelming experience.

However, overcoming these challenges and sustaining hope throughout the journey is possible.

Here are some strategies to help individuals facing cancer prevention and control:

EDUCATION AND AWARENESS:

Education and awareness play a vital role in cancer prevention and control. By providing individuals with relevant information about the causes, risk factors, and early cancer detection methods, we empower them to take proactive steps towards prevention.

One aspect of education involves educating individuals about lifestyle choices that minimize their risk of developing cancer. This includes promoting healthy habits such as regular exercise, a balanced diet, avoiding tobacco and excessive alcohol consumption, and practicing safe sun exposure. The dissemination of accurate and evidence-based information empowers individuals to make informed decisions that reduce their cancer risk.

Education is essential in raising awareness about the importance of cancer screenings and early detection. Encouraging individuals to undergo regular screenings, such as mammograms, colonoscopies, and Pap smears, can lead to the identification of cancer at its earliest stages when treatment is most effective. Education can address common misconceptions and fears surrounding these screenings, allowing individuals to overcome barriers and prioritize their health.

Furthermore, education and awareness campaigns can debunk myths and misinformation about cancer prevention and treatment. By offering scientifically accurate information, individuals can make more informed decisions about their health and seek appropriate medical care when needed.

Awareness campaigns can also focus on the importance of cancer screening and early detection. By educating individuals about the various screening methods available for different types of cancer, we can encourage them to undergo regular check-ups.

Education can help individuals recognize common cancer symptoms, enabling them to seek medical attention as soon as possible.

BUILDING A SUPPORT SYSTEM:

A support system is a crucial strategy to help individuals facing cancer prevention and control. When dealing with a potentially life-threatening illness, having a network of supportive individuals can provide emotional, practical, and informational assistance.

Emotional support plays a vital role in coping with the challenges of cancer prevention and control. Friends, family, and support groups can offer a safe space to express fears, anxieties, and frustrations. They can lend a listening ear, provide empathy, and offer encouragement, which helps individuals feel understood and validated in their struggles. This emotional support can boost resilience and motivate individuals to adhere to recommended preventative measures, psychological wellbeing, and overall treatment outcomes.

A support system can help individuals in their cancer prevention and control journey. This assistance might include helping with transportation to medical appointments, cooking meals, household chores, or caring for children. These practical tasks can alleviate the burden of daily responsibilities and enable individuals to focus on practicing healthy habits, attending screenings, and following medical advice.

Additionally, a support system can serve as a valuable source of information. Friends, family, and support groups can share knowledge about cancer prevention strategies, such as maintaining a healthy lifestyle, undergoing regular screenings, and managing risk factors. They can also provide insights and experiences regarding treatment options, healthcare providers, and support services available in the community. This information helps individuals make informed decisions and navigate the complex cancer prevention and control world more effectively.

EMBRACING MINDFULNESS AND SELF-CARE:

Mindfulness practices promote a deep sense of awareness and presence, allowing individuals to stay grounded in the present moment. This can help to alleviate anxiety and fear associated with the diagnosis, as well as reduce stress levels. By focusing on the present, individuals can better manage their emotions and cultivate a positive mindset, which is crucial for their overall mental health.

Moreover, practicing self-care is essential for individuals facing cancer prevention and control. This involves intentionally prioritizing and nurturing one's physical, mental, and emotional health. Regular exercise, healthy eating, getting enough rest, and maintaining social connections can contribute to a stronger immune system and improve overall health outcomes.

Self-care practices also give individuals a sense of agency and control over their wellbeing. By actively participating in their care, cancer patients can enhance their quality of life and regain some control amidst the uncertainty that comes with the disease.

Furthermore, incorporating mindfulness into self-care activities can enhance its benefits. Engaging in mindful eating, for example, can help individuals develop a healthier relationship with food, improve digestion, and strengthen the mind-body connection.

Similarly, mindfulness meditation can reduce treatment-related side effects such as pain, fatigue, and nausea by redirecting attention away from discomfort and fostering a sense of calm and acceptance.

SEEKING PROFESSIONAL HELP:

Healthcare professionals have the knowledge and expertise to guide individuals on cancer prevention. They can provide information on lifestyle choices, such as maintaining a healthy diet, exercising regularly, and avoiding tobacco and alcohol, which can significantly reduce the risk of developing cancer. They can offer guidance on screenings and early detection methods, ensuring that individuals are proactive in identifying potential issues.

Furthermore, professionals can help individuals navigate the emotional and psychological challenges associated with cancer prevention and control. Receiving a cancer diagnosis or undergoing treatment can be overwhelming and lead to anxiety, depression, and overall distress. Seeking professional help, such as counseling or therapy, can provide a safe space for individuals to express their feelings, cope with the diagnosis, and develop effective strategies for managing stress and maintaining mental wellbeing.

Professionals can offer support in making informed decisions regarding cancer treatment options. They can provide individuals with the most up-to-date information on various treatment modalities, including their benefits, side effects, and potential outcomes. Having a healthcare professional to discuss these options can empower individuals to make the best decisions for their circumstances.

TAKING IT ONE DAY AT A TIME:

Cancer can often feel overwhelming and uncertain. Still, by focusing on the present moment, individuals can alleviate some of the stress and anxiety associated with the disease.

Individuals can set small, achievable goals that contribute to their overall health and wellbeing by taking each day as it comes. This can include adopting healthy habits such as maintaining a balanced diet, exercising regularly, getting enough rest, and managing stress.

Moreover, taking it one day at a time allows individuals to understand and process their emotions fully. It is normal for cancer patients to experience a range of emotions, including fear, sadness, anger, and uncertainty. By acknowledging and addressing these emotions daily, individuals can develop coping mechanisms and seek the appropriate support from friends, family, and healthcare professionals.

Another benefit of approaching cancer prevention and control one day at a time is adapting and adjusting to changing circumstances. Cancer treatment plans and prognosis can often be unpredictable, so individuals need to remain flexible and open to adjusting their goals and strategies as necessary.

Taking it one day at a time can provide individuals with a renewed sense of hope and positivity. Individuals can maintain a positive outlook and increase their overall resilience by focusing on the present moment and celebrating small victories.

CELEBRATING MILESTONES:

These milestones can range from personal achievements such as completing a round of treatment, reaching a specific health goal, or simply having a good day, recognizing and acknowledging these achievements can provide a sense of encouragement and optimism.

We can foster a sense of accomplishment and positivity by acknowledging and celebrating these milestones with patients, survivors, caregivers, healthcare professionals, and the community. This enhances the emotional wellbeing of those facing cancer and boosts morale, inspiration, and determination to continue taking proactive steps towards prevention and control.

Celebrating milestones can take various forms, such as organizing events, ceremonies, or gatherings designated to honor and recognize these achievements. It can also involve highlighting individual success stories through social media, newsletters, or other communication channels to inspire and motivate others.

Moreover, celebrating milestones provides an opportunity to raise awareness about the importance of cancer prevention and control. Public recognition of achievements can generate increased interest, participation, and support from the community, leading to further advancements and progress in cancer prevention and control efforts.

Overall, overcoming challenges and sustaining hope in the cancer prevention and control journey requires a combination of education, support, self-care, goal setting, and a positive mindset. By implementing these strategies, individuals can navigate the journey resiliently and maintain hope.

CHAPTER 5

❖THRIVING IN SURVIVORSHIP

Thriving in survivorship means living well after a difficult or life-threatening experience, such as surviving cancer, a natural disaster, or any other traumatic event. It is about moving beyond survival and finding ways to heal, grow, and build a meaningful and fulfilling life.

Thriving in survivorship after cancer involves taking proactive steps to regain physical, emotional, and mental well-being.

Here are some strategies for thriving in survivorship:

HEALTH MAINTENANCE AND FOLLOW-UP CARE: Surviving cancer is a significant accomplishment, but it also comes with ongoing challenges and uncertainties. Adopting a proactive approach to health maintenance can help individuals in survivorship lead healthier lives and minimize the risk of cancer recurrence or developing other health complications.

Regularly scheduled follow-up appointments with healthcare providers are crucial for monitoring any potential signs of cancer recurrence or new cancers. These appointments typically involve physical exams, blood tests, imaging studies, and other tests as needed, depending on the individual's specific cancer history and treatment. By regularly monitoring their health, survivors and their healthcare teams can detect issues early, allowing prompt interventions and better treatment outcomes.

In addition to regular follow-up care, survivors should also engage in various self-care practices to improve their overall well-being. They should strive to maintain a healthy lifestyle by eating a balanced diet, engaging in regular physical activity, and getting sufficient restorative sleep. These factors can help manage or reduce the risk of cancer-related side effects like fatigue, weight gain, and reduced bone strength.

Furthermore, survivors may need to be diligent in managing the potential long-term effects of cancer treatment. These effects can include hormonal imbalances, heart or lung problems, or psychological issues such as anxiety and depression. Taking prescribed medications, attending therapy sessions as recommended, and seeking support from support groups or mental health professionals are crucial steps to address these challenges.

Health maintenance also involves:

- Adopting healthy habits such as quitting smoking.
- Limiting alcohol consumption.
- Avoiding exposure to environmental toxins.

Survivors should be aware of potential risk factors and take appropriate precautions to reduce their exposure to carcinogens, thus minimizing the likelihood of developing a new cancer or cancer recurrence.

Additionally, survivors should prioritize their emotional well-being and mental health. After cancer treatment, many individuals experience anxiety, fear of recurrence, or even emotional trauma. Engaging in self-care activities like mindfulness exercises and meditation or participating in supportive survivorship programs can help manage stress, improve emotional resilience, and enhance overall quality of life.

MENTAL AND EMOTIONAL WELL-BEING: Cancer can profoundly impact a person's mental and emotional state. The trauma of diagnosis, treatment, and fear of recurrence may lead to anxiety, depression, and cognitive difficulties. Therefore, it is necessary to prioritize mental and emotional well-being to support one's overall quality of life in survivorship.

One strategy for thriving in survivorship after cancer is seeking professional help. A mental health professional can provide guidance, support, and coping strategies to address the emotional toll of cancer. Therapy can assist in managing anxiety, depression, and PTSD symptoms that may arise during survivorship.

Another key aspect is establishing a strong support system. Surrounding oneself with understanding family, friends, and fellow survivors can provide empathy, encouragement, and a safe space to express emotions. Support groups, both in-person and online, allow individuals to connect with those who have had similar experiences and share valuable insights.

Taking care of physical health is also vital for mental and emotional well-being. Regular exercise, healthy eating habits, and sufficient sleep can positively impact one's mood and energy levels. Engage in stress-reducing activities such as mindfulness, meditation, or hobbies that bring joy and relaxation.

These practices can help alleviate fatigue symptoms and promote a sense of well-being.

Implementing stress management techniques is crucial. Incorporating mindfulness practices, such as meditation or deep breathing exercises, can reduce stress and enhance emotional resilience. Engaging in activities that bring joy and relaxation, such as hobbies, art, or nature walks, can also help foster a positive mindset.

Staying informed and involved in one's healthcare decisions is empowering. Individuals can regain control over their health by educating oneself about the potential long-term effects of treatment and advocating for necessary support and follow-up care.

GRADUAL RETURN TO WORK AND DAILY ACTIVITIES: It is important to acknowledge that transitioning from treatment to the post-cancer phase can pose various physical, emotional, and practical challenges.

Returning to work or resuming daily activities can promote a sense of normalcy, boost self-esteem, and provide a framework for rebuilding a fulfilling life after cancer. However, it is crucial to approach this process gradually and with self-care in mind.

In the initial stages, it is vital to prioritize self-care, listen to your body's needs, and ensure you have adequate support from healthcare professionals, friends, and family.

Consulting with your medical team about the best time to start working or engaging in daily activities is essential, as they can guide you based on your individual recovery and treatment plan.

Discussing potential modifications or accommodations at the workplace with your employer or human resources department may be helpful. This can ensure a smooth transition back to work, such as flexible working hours, reduced workload, or modified duties to accommodate any lingering physical or mental effects of cancer treatment.

Engaging in daily activities outside of work, such as hobbies, exercise, or socializing, can also contribute to your overall well-being during the survivorship phase. However, it is crucial to pace yourself and gradually increase your activity level. Remember that your body may have undergone significant changes during treatment, and it may take time to rebuild strength and endurance.

Additionally, seeking support from fellow cancer survivors, support groups, or counseling services can be extremely beneficial. They can provide a safe space to share experiences, learn coping strategies, and receive emotional support.

HEALTHY RELATIONSHIPS: Healthy relationships provide emotional support and understanding, essential during the post-cancer journey. Friends, family, or partners who can empathize and help a loving presence survivors navigate through physical and emotional challenges. Foster positive relationships with loved ones, friends, and support networks. Surround yourself with compassionate, understanding individuals who can support emotionally during challenging times.

Open and honest communication is key to any healthy relationship. This is particularly important for survivors, as they may have specific needs, concerns, or fears related to their cancer experience.

Being able to express these feelings and have someone listen and respond empathetically builds trust and strengthens the bond.

Healthy relationships provide a source of motivation and encouragement. Having loved ones who believe in the survivor's ability to overcome obstacles and pursue their goals can significantly impact their overall wellness and quality of life. Positive reinforcement helps survivors stay focused and resilient, boosting their physical and mental well-being.

Engaging in shared activities or hobbies with loved ones helps survivors regain a sense of normalcy and joy in life. These experiences can provide a much-needed distraction from the challenges of survivorship and foster a sense of connection, fostering a feeling of belonging and happiness.

Healthy relationships involve individuals willing to advocate for the survivor's needs and provide a strong support system. This may include accompanying the survivor to medical appointments, helping navigate healthcare systems, or offering practical assistance during recovery. This support can greatly reduce stress and enhance the survivor's coping ability.

Respecting the survivor's boundaries and allowing them to take control of their life post-cancer is crucial. Each survivor's experience is unique and may have specific needs or preferences regarding their health, privacy, or emotional well-being. Healthy relationships understand and honor these boundaries, ensuring the survivor's autonomy and sense of self.

CELEBRATE MILESTONES AND ACHIEVEMENTS: This practice allows individuals to acknowledge their progress and accomplishments, fostering a positive mindset and promoting overall well-being. By recognizing milestones, survivors can gain a sense of empowerment, resilience, and motivation to continue moving forward.

Celebrations can take various forms, from small gatherings with loved ones to personal rituals or self-reflection. It is crucial to honor the journey and acknowledge the challenges faced along the way. Recognizing the milestones achieved during cancer survivorship, such as completing treatment, reaching remission, or returning to daily activities, helps survivors feel fulfilled and grateful for the progress made. Recognizing and celebrating milestones can help individuals shift their focus from the hardships of cancer to the positive outcomes achieved. It allows survivors to reflect on progress, appreciate the support received, and express gratitude for every small victory. This mindset shift can contribute to a positive outlook and improved mental health.

Celebrations also allow sharing experiences with others on a similar journey. Individuals can find support, encouragement, and inspiration by connecting with fellow survivors. This sense of community can be invaluable in navigating the survivorship phase, creating lasting bonds, and expanding support networks.

Celebrating milestones provides hope and inspiration to others who may be going through similar experiences. By openly acknowledging and sharing achievements, survivors can encourage and empower others still navigating the hurdles of cancer treatment. It sends a message of resilience, determination, and optimism, fostering a supportive environment for all.

Furthermore, celebrating milestones and achievements can serve as a reminder of one's resilience and strength. Cancer survivorship can be physically, emotionally, and mentally demanding.

Recognizing and celebrating progress promotes self-confidence and self-belief, reinforcing the survivor's ability to overcome difficult situations.

ENGAGE IN SURVIVORSHIP PROGRAMS/RESOURCES: Engaging in survivorship programs and resources can be an effective strategy for thriving in survivorship after cancer. These programs and resources are designed to support individuals who have completed cancer treatment and help them transition into their new normal.

Survivorship programs provide education and tools to help individuals understand and manage the physical and emotional challenges that may arise after cancer treatment. Through workshops, classes, and support groups, survivors can learn coping skills, stress management techniques, and self-care strategies to improve their well-being.

Survivorship programs offer opportunities for survivors to connect with others who have had similar experiences. This sense of community and understanding can be incredibly valuable as survivors navigate the unique challenges they may face. Sharing stories, encouraging, and exchanging advice with others who have been through cancer can foster a sense of hope and resilience.

Furthermore, survivorship programs provide access to various resources and services that can address specific needs post-cancer. These resources may include nutrition counseling, rehabilitation services, financial assistance, and career guidance. By utilizing these resources, survivors can overcome barriers that may hinder their ability to thrive personally and professionally.

Engaging in survivorship programs and resources helps individuals navigate the challenges of survivorship and empowers them to take an active role in their own well-being. By being proactive about their health and actively seeking support, survivors can optimize their physical and emotional recovery, enhance their quality of life, and find a renewed sense of purpose and resilience in their survivorship journey.

Take advantage of survivorship programs, support groups, and resources from cancer centers or local organizations. These programs provide educational resources, peer support, and networking opportunities, fostering community and empowerment.

ADVOCACY AND GIVING BACK: Advocacy and giving back can be crucial in helping individuals thrive in survivorship after cancer. By actively engaging in advocacy efforts, survivors not only contribute to raising awareness about cancer but also empower themselves and others affected by the disease.

Advocacy involves speaking out for change, whether it be through sharing personal experiences, supporting policy initiatives, or promoting research advancements. By using their journey with cancer, survivors can drive understanding, acceptance, and empathy among the general public. This helps reduce stigma and encourages early detection, prompt treatment, and overall improved outcomes for future cancer patients.

Moreover, engaging in advocacy can enable survivors to reclaim their sense of purpose and control in life after cancer. It provides a platform for them to make a difference and effect positive change in the cancer community. Through advocacy, survivors can find renewed strength and a sense of meaning, shifting the focus from being a victim to becoming a survivor and a proactive agent of change.

In addition to advocacy, giving back is another strategy that can greatly contribute to thriving in survivorship. Giving back can take various forms, such as volunteering time or resources to cancer organizations, supporting fellow survivors, or participating in fundraisers or awareness events. Survivors can find fulfillment, gratitude, and a deeper connection to the cancer community by giving back.

Contributing to the well-being of others affected by cancer can foster a sense of unity and support among survivors. It creates an environment of shared experiences and underscores the belief that no one should face cancer alone. This camaraderie can provide emotional healing, social support, and a sense of belonging.

Furthermore, giving back allows survivors to channel their energy and emotions towards a positive cause, which may help alleviate any lingering anxiety, fear, or sadness associated with their cancer journey.

By helping others, survivors can find solace in knowing that they are making a difference in someone else's life and, in turn, find a renewed sense of purpose and hope in their own.

By sharing your story and providing support, you can make a positive impact on the lives of others and find meaning in your journey.

CONCLUSION

The conclusion of the book titled "Defeating the Silent Invader (Cancer): Building a Stronger Immune System and Overcoming Cancer's Survival Tactics with the Right Diet and Lifestyle Choices" emphasizes the importance of taking a comprehensive approach to battling cancer. Throughout the book, the author has provided evidence-based information about how a strong immune system and healthy lifestyle choices can play a crucial role in overcoming cancer.

By adopting the right diet and lifestyle choices, individuals can strengthen their immune system, making it more effective in targeting and eliminating cancer cells.

The book highlighted the importance of consuming a balanced diet rich in fruits, vegetables, whole grains, and lean proteins while minimizing the intake of processed foods, high-sugar items, and unhealthy fats.

Moreover, the author stressed the significance of maintaining a physically active lifestyle and managing stress through meditation and exercise. These practices contribute to a healthier overall well-being and enhance the immune system's ability to recognize and fight against cancer cells.

The book also highlighted the importance of early detection and regular medical check-ups. It emphasized the need for individuals to proactively understand their bodies, recognize potential warning signs, and seek professional medical advice promptly.

"Defeating the Silent Invader (Cancer)" encourages readers to take charge of their health by making informed and conscious lifestyle choices. By nurturing a strong immune system, adopting a healthy diet, staying physically active, managing stress, and seeking appropriate medical care, individuals can significantly boost their chances of overcoming cancer and leading healthier lives.

Building a Stronger Immune System and Overcoming Cancer's Survival Tactics with the Right Diet and Lifestyle Choices" emphasizes the significance of adopting a holistic approach to cancer treatment.

It highlights the power of a strong immune system and how it can effectively combat cancer cells.

The book presents numerous scientifically-backed studies and anecdotal evidence, showcasing the undeniable connection between a healthy lifestyle, proper nutrition, and cancer prevention. The conclusion compiles this information and stresses the importance of incorporating specific diet and lifestyle choices into one's daily routine.

Regular physical activity is also highlighted as a crucial part of maintaining a strong immune system. The book suggests incorporating moderate exercise into daily routines, such as brisk walks, yoga, or strength training, to enhance overall health and well-being.

Additionally, the conclusion draws attention to the detrimental effects of smoking, excessive alcohol consumption, and exposure to environmental toxins on the immune system and cancer development. It encourages readers to eliminate or minimize these harmful habits to reduce their cancer risk.

The book concludes by emphasizing the importance of regular medical check-ups, screenings, and early cancer detection. It promotes a proactive approach to healthcare, urging readers to seek medical advice and guidance to ensure early intervention if the need arises.

Ultimately, the conclusion of "Defeating the Silent Invader (Cancer)" provides readers with the knowledge and tools to make informed decisions about their diet, lifestyle choices, and overall health. It emphasizes the power of a strong immune system and how it can be crucial in defeating cancer and improving overall well-being.